Apple Cider Vinegar
For Natural Health

Ellen Vincent

First Printing, 2012

ISBN-13: 978-1475220704

ISBN-10: 1475220707

Printed in the United States of America

Dedication

For my son Titus

Apple Cider Vinegar

For Natural Health

Table of Contents

Introduction

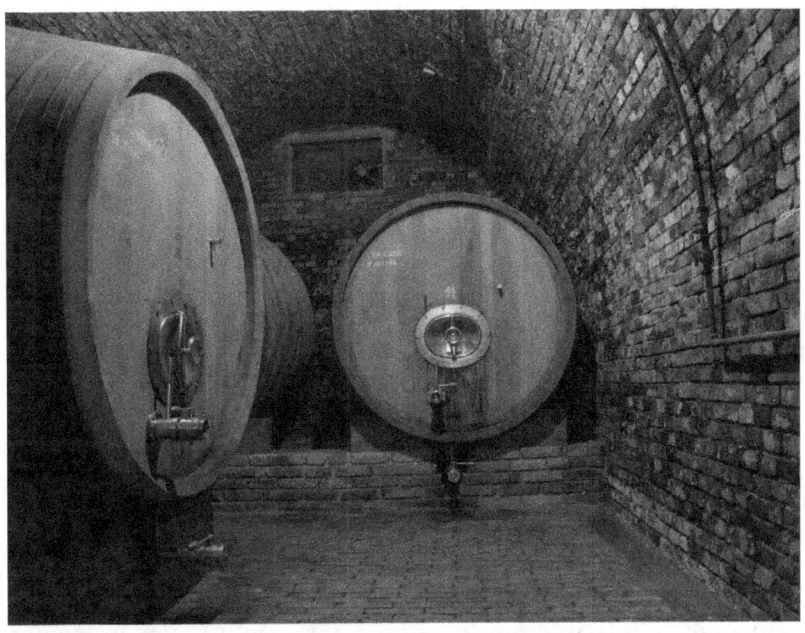

Vinegar has proved to be a useful substance over the years and has been used as the solution for many problems. One of the main uses has been in the preservation of food. Before we had freezers, food preservation was a real problem and vinegar was and still is an important food preservative. We have all come across pickles whether it be pickled onions or Dill pickles. These food items are put into vinegar and then put into jars. These will then keep fresh because the vinegar prevents the growth of micro organisms which would usually make these foods go off over time. Modern pickled onions should be the same but I suspect these days that vinegar may just be added to the jars for flavoring rather than as a preservative. Other uses for vinegar included cleaning in the home, polishing metals and killing weeds. I regularly use vinegar to clean windows and mirrors where it can remove dirt as well as all those annoying smears. Vinegar is also used extensively in the preparation of foods such as salad dressings, some curries and sweet and sour dishes.

Apple cider vinegar is a totally natural product. However, you should be aware that other vinegars may be produced by chemical means and these are not considered to be natural products at all. This type of vinegar is referred to as non brewed condiment and is often used in Fish and Chip shops in the UK. Apple cider vinegar on the other hand is simply cider that has gone off. We all know that leaving a bottle of wine open will cause it to go off and have a bitter taste. This is the bitter taste of the vinegar as it forms in the wine from the alcohol. This is because vinegar bacteria get into the wine and cause it to change the alcohol in it into the substance that we know as vinegar. In the same way vinegar bacteria get into cider and then make that change into vinegar. Vinegar is an acid. The acid is weak and of the same nature as lemon juice. These weak acids can be used in food because they won't cause any harm to the human body. This is in contrast to strong acids such as those in car batteries which are very corrosive and will even burn the skin if they get onto it. Although vinegar doesn't burn you can certainly feel it stinging if it gets into any cuts on your hands and fingers or the eyes. The acid in vinegar is called acetic acid and has a different structure to the weak citric acid found in fruits such as lemons and oranges.

The important basic fact about apple cider vinegar is that it comes from apples. As stated earlier vinegar can be made from any other alcoholic drinks and as such you will more than likely have come across wine vinegar and the more common malt vinegar. I guess you could consider malt vinegar as beer that has gone off. Because apple cider vinegar is based on apples it means that all of the other nutrients from the apples are still present in the vinegar and this includes minerals, vitamins, anti oxidants, fruit acids and amino acids. It is this combination of different nutrients as well as the vinegar element itself which comes into play when considering any health benefits of using apple cider vinegar.

The healing effects of apple cider vinegar have been known for centuries and it has been used by our ancient ancestor's right through until the present time. A lot of these remedies have entered into folklore but this doesn't mean that they shouldn't be taken seriously. The more we understand about the chemical makeup of apple cider vinegar the more we should take its value seriously. For a start of, the various acids and minerals that are found in it can help to keep the balance of acids in the body steady. Minerals are needed in the various chemical reactions in the body that keep us alive. These reactions are referred to as metabolism. There are up to 20 minerals in apple cider vinegar and these include potassium, phosphorus, magnesium, calcium, chlorine and sulfur. There are also up to a 100 other chemical compounds in it, which are all important for metabolism in the body. It is thought that this array of different substances is the reason that apple cider vinegar has found importance in helping with a number of health conditions such as weight management, heart disease, diabetes, fighting infection, arthritis and osteoporosis. This book tries to explain where apple cider vinegar can help us to maintain our health and how best to use it from day to day.

The treatments in this book are ones that have been used for centuries and are therefore referred to as folk remedies. Where as there is a lot of anecdotal evidence about their success, there is very little solid scientific research to back any of it up. As a result you should only try them if you think you would like to find out if they are good for you. It is really proposed that you might use apple cider vinegar in addition to other treatments for a particular condition rather than just relying on it on its own. If you are taking medicines prescribed by your doctor you certainly shouldn't stop taking them in favor of using apple cider vinegar instead. When considering the use of apple cider vinegar for a medical condition always consult your doctor first.

I regularly use apple cider vinegar to treat my dandruff and I now swear by it. I have also tried it on my athlete's foot and found that the itchiness and pain just melt away. My husband and I are off to a local apple farm on Sunday to pick up a few gallons of the 'good stuff' to keep me going. This is far cheaper and better quality than anything you are going to get in a health food shop!

The remedies described are for the use of adults. You shouldn't use apple cider vinegar with children unless you have the clearance of your doctor.

There are some conditions for which apple cider vinegar has been proposed but, when you look into it, the evidence really isn't there to support its use. One such condition is the treatment of genital warts. This seems to be something that has been propagated by the internet as some kind of urban myth. As a result, if there is some doubt about the usefulness of apple cider vinegar for a particular condition you should make sure that you research the evidence and consult professional advice as well.

Raw apple cider vinegar

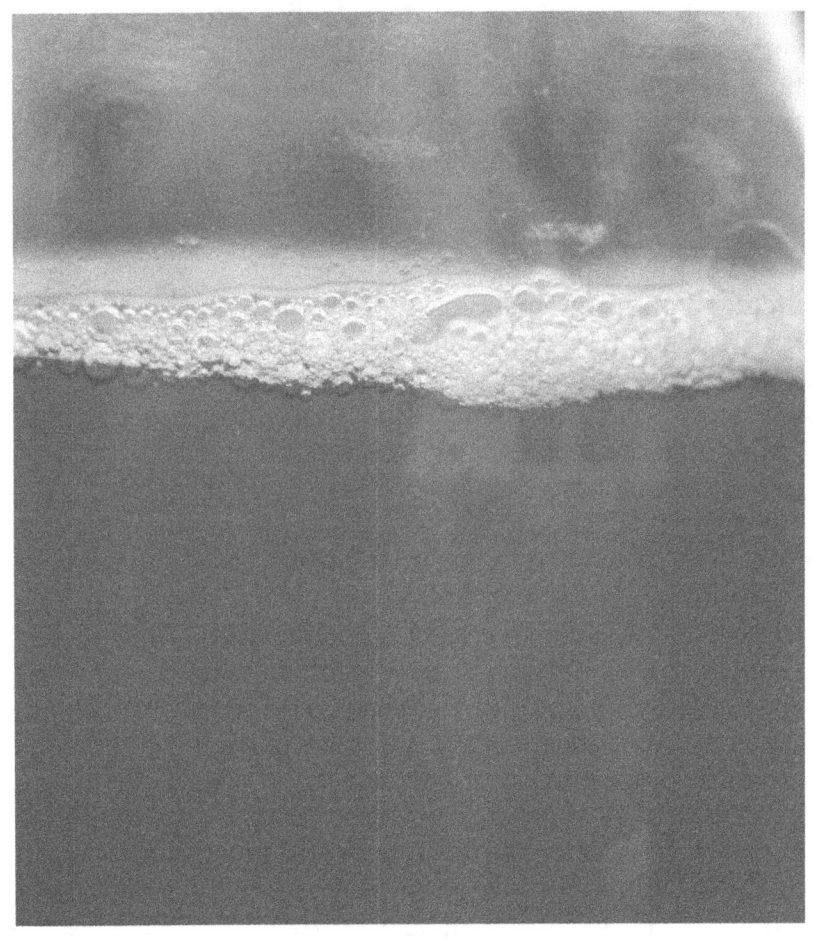

Raw apple cider vinegar contains more than just acetic acid and it looks different to the stuff you can buy in supermarkets and health shops. This raw material is to be found in farm shops operated by cider farmers. They simply put some of their cider to one side; cover it up with muslin cloth to stop insects getting in; and leave it for some months for the vinegar to develop. The cloth allows oxygen to get to the cider. This is important, because oxygen is needed for the vinegar bacteria to work. The vinegar bacteria collect on the surface of the cider and do their work converting the alcohol in the cider into vinegar. This process relies on wild bacteria getting into the cider. To help the process along, some farmers will have kept bacteria from previous batches that have produced good vinegar. They then add this collection of bacteria or 'vinegar mother' to the cider and this gets the process to start a lot faster.

You can buy apple cider vinegar with the 'vinegar mother' included and some people say that this is the best form of it to use for treating health problems and as a tonic to keep the body healthy. The raw cider and mother will contain a lot more natural fiber, enzymes, proteins and amino acids compared to the filtered clear and pasteurized bottles that are on supermarket shelves.

You can also make your own apple cider vinegar by following a similar process. Leave cider in a jug exposed to the air but covered with muslin cloth. After a few months natural bacteria in the environment will have changed the alcohol into vinegar. The results might not be as good as that from a big farm producer but this is certainly something that you can try for yourself. If you get a batch of homemade vinegar that is to your liking save the mother from the top of the vinegar and use it again in your next batch. Alternatively you could ask a cider farmer for some of the mother that they use or simply use some of the raw cider vinegar that you buy as a starter. If you are doing this you must make sure that the vinegar hasn't been pasteurized as the mother will have been destroyed in the process.

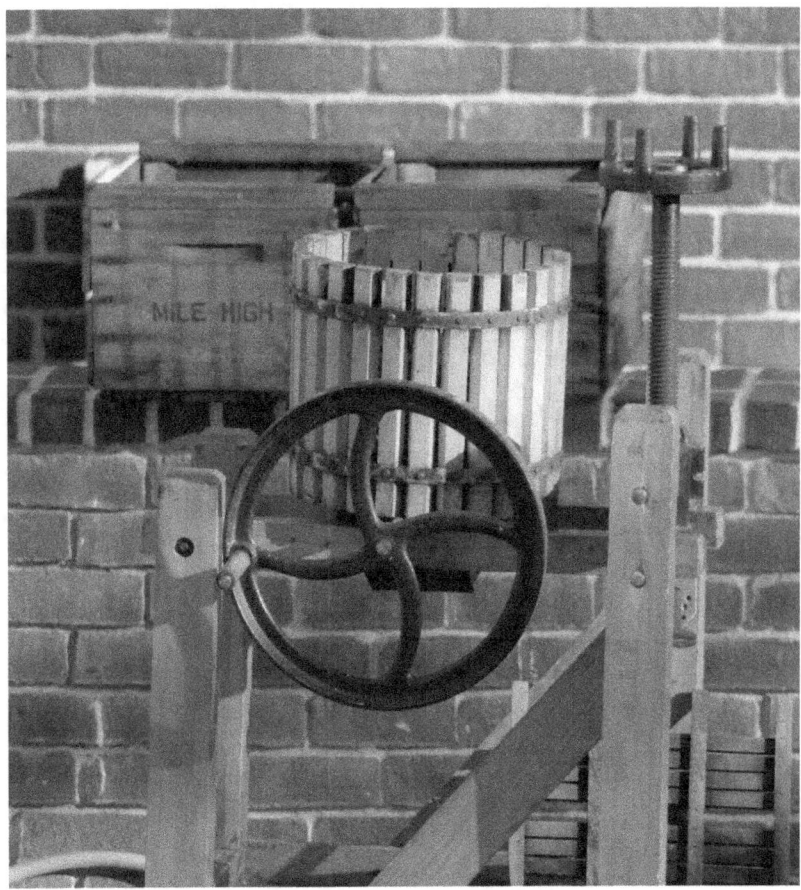

Diabetes

People with diabetes have problems with maintaining their blood sugar levels. Normally blood sugar is kept under control under the influence of the hormone insulin, which makes the liver convert glucose into the storage compound glycogen when the level of glucose in the blood increases above normal. High glucose levels in the blood are a problem because they make the cells of the body lose water and this causes them problems in performing their usual metabolic activities. Cells such as those of the nervous system are very sensitive to glucose levels in the blood.

Type 1 diabetes is a life long condition and starts when people are young due to an infection. People with type 1 diabetes need to take insulin on a regular basis. Type 2 diabetes affects older people and often occurs in people who have problems with obesity. These people can become resistant to the affects of insulin and as a result the insulin in the body isn't as effective at reducing blood sugar levels as it should be. People who are slightly resistant to insulin can be identified before the onset of diabetes. These people are referred to as being pre-diabetic. Pre-diabetes and even milder forms of diabetes can often be reversed by addressing life style issues such as obesity.

People can suffer from different severities of type 2 diabetes. In the most severe cases diabetics have to inject themselves with insulin, if their blood sugar levels rise too much. Other people with less severe forms can often control their blood sugar levels by being careful with their diet. Such things as avoiding very sugary foods and avoiding having large meals with large gaps between without eating can help. Other people have to take tablets to control their blood sugar levels. These tablets often have side effects which can make life more of a challenge by increasing tiredness and making people more lethargic and less able to get on with their normal lives.

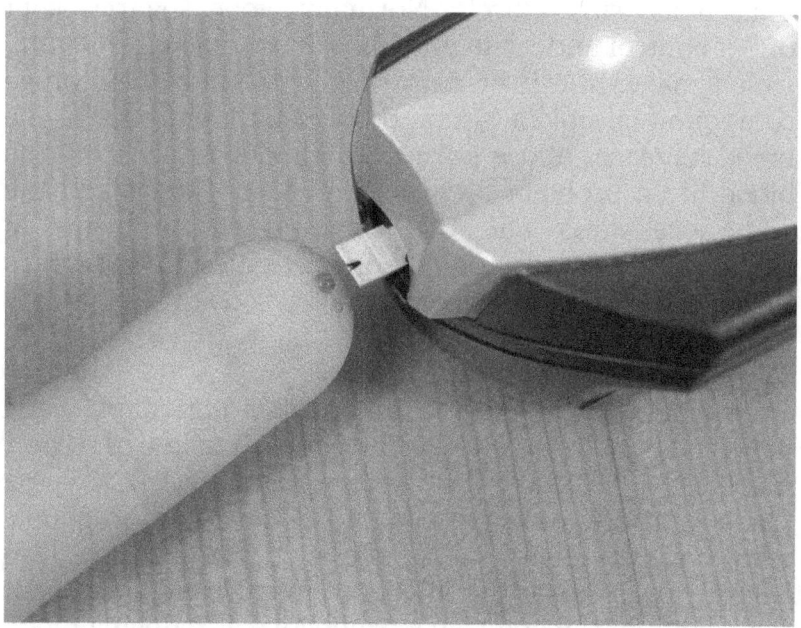

It stands to reason that any natural substances that can lower blood sugar levels without causing side effects would be a real bonus. Apple cider vinegar is reported to be just such a natural ingredient. There has been quite a lot of research in the ability of apple cider vinegar to reduce the blood sugar levels in people suffering from diabetes.

Studies at Arizona State University concentrated on giving apple cider vinegar to subjects at particular times of the day and then comparing the test group with a control group that were given only a placebo drink.

In the first study, apple cider vinegar was given to the subjects before they had their regular meal. The subjects were made up of equal numbers of people with type 2 diabetes, pre-diabetes and a group that didn't have diabetes at all. There were approximately 30 people in total involved in the study. Before a high carbohydrate breakfast of orange juice and a bagel half of the group was given 4 teaspoons of apple cider vinegar. The other half of the group were given a placebo drink which didn't contain vinegar. A week later the roles of the placebo and test group were reversed in what is called a cross over trial. Blood sugar levels in the subjects were tested after the meal. It was found that the rise in blood sugar level in all three groups was slower than one would have expected compared to the control placebo group. In the case of the pre-diabetics blood sugar levels were 34% lower and in the type 2 diabetes group 19% lower. It is thought that the apple cider vinegar reduces the absorption of digested carbohydrate from the gut after the meal. This then leads to the reduction in carbohydrate levels in the blood. It is interesting to note that this is the way that Acarbose and Metformin diabetes medicines work when they are prescribed for the diabetes condition. Apple cider vinegar, however, is completely natural and has no side effects

In a second study apple cider vinegar was given before bedtime. Eleven people were involved in the study and they all had the early stages of type 2 diabetes. This means that their condition was treated with tablets rather than insulin injections. Before bedtime the individuals were either given cheese and 2 tablespoons of apple cider vinegar or cheese and water. This procedure was repeated for 2 days. After a few more days the vinegar and placebo water group were crossed over and the trial repeated. In the mornings after each trial the individuals involved had their fasting blood sugar concentrations tested. The study found that the apple cider vinegar group had fasting glucose levels that were on average 2% lower than the placebo group taking the water instead of vinegar. These results are encouraging and show that apple cider vinegar can bring about a significant drop in blood sugar levels over night, in people with mild type 2 diabetes.

A further study was conducted on 30 healthy adults to see what effect taking apple cider vinegar would have on blood sugar levels after a meal. After overnight fasting the group were given a meal consisting of a bagel with butter and fruit juice. Again they were either given 2 teaspoons of vinegar or water as a placebo. Two hours after having the meal the trial group had their glucose blood levels tested. It was found that the group taking the apple cider vinegar had a reduced glucose blood level of 20% when compared to those that had consumed the placebo water in place of the vinegar. This is significant when you consider that diabetics are recommended to take procedures to reduce their blood sugar levels after a meal in order to avoid complications that can be caused by the diabetes condition. Further studies have determined that the most effective dose of vinegar involves 2 teaspoons of apple cider vinegar that contains 5% of acetic acid. It has also been found that it is better to take the vinegar with the meal rather than after it. Based on this the vinegar could be taken in hot tea with lemon with the meal. It is feared that 20% of American adults could be suffering from some form of diabetes in the next few years and as a result apple cider vinegar could be one way that people could self treat themselves in the early stages of pre-diabetes without suffering any of the side effects caused by the prescribed drugs that are currently used to treat diabetes.

High cholesterol

Cholesterol in the blood stream has been pin pointed as one of the main factors involved in the deposition of the fatty plaque like material in arteries that is responsible for coronary heart disease. There are in fact two types of cholesterol found in the blood. Only one of them appears to be responsible for the fatty deposits on artery walls. This particular one is called Low Density Lipoprotein or LDL cholesterol. The other type is called High Density Lipoprotein or HDL cholesterol. HDL cholesterol appears to have a beneficial effect and can protect the body against the build up of these fatty deposits. Both types of cholesterol are important for the normal working of the body and are involved in cell division and dealing with stress. To this end the liver produces enough of each type of cholesterol to keep the body in tip top condition. As a result there is in fact little need to get extra cholesterol in the foods that we eat. The liver tries to maintain a normal ratio of about 4 parts HDL to 10 parts LDL. If the ratio falls below 3 parts to 10 then that is when the extra LDL causes its bad effects on the body. As the ratio decreases more and more lipoprotein is deposited in the artery walls. If these plaques become too large they can restrict the flow of blood in the artery. This is very dangerous if these deposits are in the thin coronary arteries that supply food and oxygen to the heart itself. The first signs of a real problem are the pains associated with the condition known as angina. The pain is caused by the fact that the heart muscles can't get enough oxygen to fuel them during heavy exercise. Eventually the fatty deposit can block one of these thin arteries and a heart attack is the result.

As a result we need to try and keep our ratio of blood HDL to LDL as high as we can. Modern diets have made this difficult because of the huge amount of animal fats in meats and dairy products. These all contain saturated fats which give rise to more of the bad LDL cholesterol. Health advice usually advises people to reduce the amount of saturated fats that they consume. This in turn should lead to a restoration of the correct ratio of these two cholesterols. People may be given medicines called statins by their doctor. These help to reduce the amount of LDL cholesterol in the blood stream. Unfortunately they can give rise to side effects such as joint and muscle pains in a number of people. This is where apple cider vinegar comes into its own. It can also help to reduce the amount of LDL cholesterol in the body. This could be a great advantage for people who are looking a more natural way to control cholesterol levels without all of the problems of side effects caused by the usual prescribed medicines.

The main way that apple cider vinegar works to lower cholesterol levels is by preventing digested fatty foods from getting into the body from the gut. Apple cider vinegar contains a lot of the soluble fiber called pectin. This actually comes from the apples that the cider vinegar is made of. Pectin is not found in other vinegars such as those made from malt. The pectin fiber binds to fats and cholesterol in the gut and prevents it from getting into the blood stream. It is thought that the acid conditions provided by the acetic acid in the vinegar helps this binding to occur. Once the fatty materials are bound to the pectin they carry on through the gut until they are egested from the body at the other end of the digestive system. There are other water soluble pectins in apple cider vinegar which add bulk to foods and this can help to make you feel full. The net result of this is that you eat less and in particular less fatty foods such as snacks. This in turn also helps to reduce the amount of cholesterol forming fats that enter the blood stream from the gut.

There have been experiments on rats which have shown that apple cider vinegar can lower cholesterol levels when added to their diet. This however, is only an indication that a similar thing happens in humans. Despite the lack of scientific evidence most people find that consuming one tablespoon of apple cider vinegar a day can help to lower their blood cholesterol levels.

High blood pressure and heart health

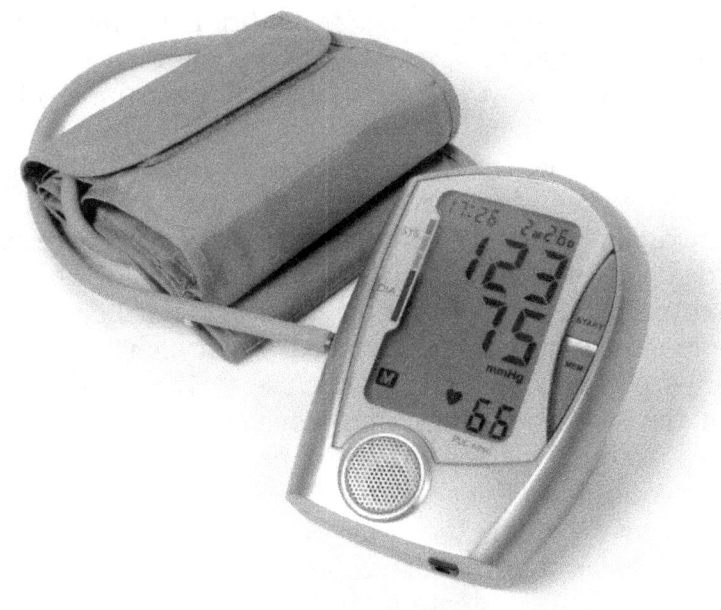

High blood pressure can cause many long term health problems. These conditions include heart attacks, strokes, congestive heart failure, kidney disease and aneurysms. These diseases tend to build up over the years and can be driven by high blood pressure which forces the blood through the blood vessels with a higher force than normal. This in turn tends to increase the deposition of fatty material onto the walls of arteries.

The whole situation is made a lot worse if the people concerned also have high blood cholesterol levels as well. There are tablets that can be prescribed by doctors for high blood pressure but these often have side effects and can lead to complications such as diabetes. As a result patients with suspected high blood pressure are often given a chance to try and reduce their own blood pressure. There are many methods that can be used such as reducing stress, reducing dietary salt, losing weight and taking regular exercise. In addition to this there is also some evidence for taking apple cider vinegar on a regular basis as a way to stabilize blood pressure levels.

Scientific studies involving rats has discovered that apple cider vinegar can lower blood pressure in those individuals where it is higher than normal. There have also been studies involving humans. One of these discovered that people eating salad dressings containing apple cider vinegar had reduced levels of heart disease compared to those who did not use it. It was important that the salad dressings were consumed at least 5 to 6 times a week for the effect to be of any significance. However, due to the general nature of the study it is still not clear whether the vinegar was the actual active ingredient or another part of the salad dressing or even a very specific combination of ingredients in the meals involved.

Using apple cider vinegar is really easy. To start off with, mix 2 teaspoons of apple cider vinegar into a pint of water and drink this each day. You should, however, be ready for the taste that you will experience. You will probably think that it isn't the most delicious flavor that you have ever experienced. However, you will soon get used to the taste and the end results on your blood pressure should certainly be worth it. If you still find the taste not to your liking you can use warm water and add a spoonful of honey. The warm water will help to mix the honey with the water and vinegar. This should definitely improve the taste. You can also try adding apple cider vinegar to extra virgin olive oil and use it as a salad dressing instead of the normal one that you use.

Cancer

There are some publications claiming that apple cider vinegar can cure cancer. There is no evidence to support this and people with cancer should rely on the drugs prescribed by their physicians rather than using or switching to apple cider vinegar.

There is however, a possibility that apple cider vinegar could help to prevent cancer to a certain extent however this is simply due to the levels of antioxidants and soluble fiber that it contains. Antioxidants are powerful natural substances which help our body's to deal with chemical agents called free radicals. These free radicals are released into the body when it comes into contact with pollutants and other poisonous chemicals in the environment. Free radicals can damage the cells of the body which can lead to aging and also cancer. Pectin is the soluble fiber in apple cider vinegar and this can help prevent colon cancer by ensuring that food doesn't lie in the colon of the digestive system for too long. However, it should be clear that apple cider vinegar will be no better at preventing these cancers when compared to other foods with high levels of antioxidants and fiber content.

Scientific research in this area has been rather confusing as far as apple cider vinegar is concerned. Some studies have suggested that consuming apple cider vinegar can help to decrease the risk of getting esophageal cancer; however, others have even produced evidence of an increase in the risk of suffering bladder cancer.

Weight loss

Vinegar has been used for centuries as a part of many different weight loss programs. It has been reported that vinegar, in general, can help people to feel full. This is quite significant when you consider that most people break their diets due to cravings for snacks and other foods because they just don't feel full when eating the food advised by their diet. A study in 2005 found that people who consumed bread along with a small amount of vinegar said that they felt more satisfied and full compared to others in the test group who consumed bread alone. This study only involved a small number of test subjects and is therefore only a tantalizing taste of what vinegar can actually do in the field of weight loss.

In another study involving obese individuals in Japan people taking vinegar each day were compared with individuals who took no vinegar at all. In the study a group of individuals with similar body masses, body mass indexes and waist circumferences were used. The individuals in the group were then either given 30ml, 15ml or 0ml of vinegar on a daily basis for 12 weeks. After this time measurements were taken of waist circumference, blood fats, body fat area, body mass and BMI. It was found that all these measurements were lower in those taking the vinegar compared to the control group taking no vinegar. None of the individuals knew whether they were taking vinegar or not. Although the overall weight losses were quite small for each vinegar taking group it was found that those taking the 30ml of vinegar did lose the most weight. It was also noted that the 2 vinegar taking groups consumed less calories when compared to the control group. As a result it was concluded that the results were probably due to a lack of appetite caused by drinking the vinegar. This study was conducted just using basic vinegar and as a result apple cider vinegar should be even better at reducing appetite due to the inclusion of pectin soluble fiber which makes the person feel fuller for longer.

Apple cider vinegar for acid reflux

Acid reflux is where the concentrated hydrochloric acid normally found in the stomach manages to leave the stomach and enters the esophagus or food pipe. A ring of muscles called a sphincter controls the movement of substances between the esophagus and the stomach. This movement should be one way from the esophagus and into the stomach. Gravity and the contraction of the circular muscles in the esophageal wall all help to propel balls of food and liquids that are drunk into the stomach. Once the food is in the stomach the sphincter muscle prevents it re-entering the esophagus. This is a good thing because the contents of the stomach are digested using strong hydrochloric acid and protein digesting enzymes. The stomach is protected against these corrosive agents by a layer of mucus.

The mucus layer in the esophagus isn't thick enough to serve as much protection against such acids. During acid reflux the acids and enzymes manage to enter the esophagus once again and here they can damage the esophageal wall. The reason for the movement into the esophagus is that the sphincter doesn't work correctly and doesn't seal the contents in the stomach. During this movement the acids can also damage the sphincter muscles even more causing the condition to get worse.

Once the acids and enzymes are in the esophagus and damaging its wall the sufferer will experience pains which are described as a burning sensation. This is often called heartburn. The condition is made worse when a person is lying down on his or her back or indulging in bending actions such as picking things up, especially if the work is hard. During this acid reflux the sphincter muscle may also get damaged further which can make the acid reflux more likely in the future. Besides causing a lot of misery and pain acid reflux can also lead to some serious conditions such as cancer of the esophagus.

Controlling acid reflux is a matter of debate but most prescribed medication involves the use of antacids which when swallowed reduce the acid levels in the stomach. This then means that there is less irritation of the sphincter muscle and less heartburn if acid reflux takes place. This situation works fine until the antacid is used up. The problem then is that the stomach may start to produce even more acid to try and increase the acidity in there for digestion to take place as normal. This can then get into a vicious circle with increasing need for antacid because of the extra acid produced.

A surprising suggestion for dealing with acid reflux is the use of apple cider vinegar. On the face of this it would seem to be a ridiculous notion that an acid problem can be dealt with by adding even more acid. However, apple cider vinegar has a number of properties that can help when compared to using antacids. To start off with the soluble fiber in apple cider vinegar will tend to absorb the digestive juices making them work more efficiently and keeping them where they are really needed in the stomach itself. The acid in stomach juices is a strong one called Hydrochloric acid where as the acid in vinegar is a weak one called acetic acid. A peculiar thing happens when weak and strong acids like these are mixed together and that is that the weaker acid tends to keep the acidity levels to a set level. In doing this they can stop the acid in the stomach getting too strong and maintain it at the level needed for digestion to be done efficiently. This mechanism is called buffering and is used throughout the body to stop tissues and fluids becoming extreme in their acidity or even alkalinity. As a result the apple cider vinegar actually reduces the possible acid levels in the stomach and this can mean less irritation to the sphincter muscle and in turn less acid reflux.

It is also thought that raw apple cider vinegar which contains the original vinegar producing material or 'vinegar mother' is far better at maintaining the acid levels than any refined or purified form of it. The reason for this is unknown, but it could be due to the rich array of minerals or the vinegar bacteria themselves that prove to be helpful.

It appears to be best to take the apple cider vinegar before meal times making sure that you shake it up to include the mother. One tablespoon should be sufficient and you can mix it with water to dilute it and make it more palatable. Alternatively mix it with mayonnaise or salad oil to use during the meal. Most people trying this method say that they get improvements in their situation as months of treatment continue

Constipation

A lot of people suffer the unnecessary pain associated with constipation. The food remains in the bowels for far too long and then it is difficult and often painful to try and get it to move out of the body. In addition to this the waste food in the bowel starts to rot if it remains there too long. This can cause the release of toxins which are believed to be able to promote such diseases as cancer. Fortunately apple cider vinegar can help to get the food moving in a more natural way. This is because it contains natural soluble fiber which helps the movement of food along the digestive system. In addition to this, the raw cider vinegar can act as a laxative which causes the muscles in the gut wall to contract and push the food further along and out of the body. Obviously, you should make sure that you add more fruit and vegetables to your diet as well as having a daily tonic of diluted apple cider vinegar.

Fighting yeast infections

Apple cider vinegar has been used for centuries to kill and prevent the growth of micro organisms. You only have to look at its use in the food preservation industry to see how good it is at dealing with the micro organisms that cause food to spoil. This whole industry has its own special name of pickling. You can also use vinegar to kill micro organisms such as bacteria and fungi on surfaces. You simply wipe over the surface you want to clean with vinegar on a cloth. Many years ago, in the times of plague, vinegar was used to prevent the plague disease from being transferred from contaminated people in plague infested villages. Food was left at the edge of the village and money was left in a pot of vinegar for the sellers so that any plague organisms were killed.

Apple cider vinegar is also very good at dealing with fungal infections. An illustration of this is its use in treating athlete's foot. This is a very well known fungal infection on the feet. The causative organism is called 'trichophyton rubrum' and it is very infectious especially when people share bathing areas and items such as towels. Once a person has athlete's foot it tends to persist unless it is treated. As with all fungi they have to have the correct conditions in order to thrive and this includes warmth and moisture. As a result the area between the toes is ideal, especially if the feet have been sweating while in socks and shoes. The sweat will change the acid balance of the skin and this can encourage the growth of fungi. In addition to this the moisture from sweat also makes the skin between the toes become soft and this more easily allows the fungal threads of the organism to infect it. Once infected and the fungus has been given a chance to develop on the skin an itchy red rash appears and then the skin becomes soft and very sensitive. Eventually the skin may peel away causing more pain and sensitivity.

Apple cider vinegar can be used to treat these raw, red and damaged areas on the feet. It will get rid of the continuous itch and can even get rid of the fungus all together. The relief is almost immediate and so, despite the smell of the vinegar itself it is really worthwhile using it. The best way to apply the apple cider vinegar is to produce a mixture to soak your feet in. To do this make a mixture of half apple cider vinegar and half warm water. Gently clean your feet with a mild soap and then soak them in the vinegar mixture for about 20 minutes. After this treatment gently clean your feet with soap and water once again. Make sure you dry your feet thoroughly so that there are no moist areas that will encourage the growth of the fungus once again. If the infection is severe than you can try soaking your feet in the apple cider mixture twice a day otherwise once a day should be sufficient. You should repeat the treatment for up to two weeks and after this time it should be gone.

If you only have a mild case of athlete's foot then it is usually sufficient to wipe over the infected area with a cloth or piece of cotton wool soaked in apple cider vinegar. As you gently rub the cloth over the affected area the itchiness is relieved.

To prevent further infections of athlete's foot you should take steps to reduce your exposure to the fungus. As with all infections, prevention is easier and better than the cure. To prevent exposure to the organism wear waterproof sandals in public bathing and shower areas. As well as this make sure that you keep your feet dry and wear socks and footwear that allow the feet to breath. Cotton or wool socks are better at providing ventilation of the feet and toes compared to man made materials. If your feet get particularly sweaty it is a good idea to change them for fresh socks during the day. You should try to wear shoes that provide ventilation and allow them to dry out between periods of wearing them.

There are other fungal infections that can benefit from being treated with apple cider vinegar and these include candidiasis, oral yeast infection, and other intestinal fungal infections. Yeast infections of the skin become apparent due to an imbalance of organisms on the skin. Usually the skin has its own natural populations of helpful bacteria. These tend to stop slower growing fungal organisms from infecting and getting a hold on the skin. However, such things as immune deficiencies and hormonal imbalances can cause the friendly bacteria to reduce in numbers and as a result they can no longer keep the yeast organisms in check. Once again apple cider vinegar can be used to deal with these yeast infections and thereby restore the natural balance of organisms on the skin. The vinegar does this because of its anti fungal and anti bacterial properties.

To deal with fungal infections on the skin you can add vinegar to your bath. Add just 2 cups of vinegar mixed with warm water to your bath and then allow yourself to soak in the bath for about 30 minutes. Make sure that the infected areas are under the water all of the time otherwise the treatment won't be effective.

Genital candidiasis can be treated by preparing douches made up of vinegar and warm water mixtures. Simply mix 2 tablespoons of the apple cider vinegar   with 2 quarts of warm water. Dip a sterile piece of cotton into the mixture and apply it to the area that is infected.

Oral thrush and gastrointestinal yeast infections can be treated by making up a drink made up of 2 or 3 teaspoons of apple cider vinegar added to about 250 ml of fresh water. If you drink this 3 times a day for about a week these fungal infections should start to ease.

If any of these conditions fail to respond to these treatments then you should definitely seek professional advice because some yeast infections may be an indication of a more serious imbalance within the body caused by a more serious condition.

The apple cider vinegar cold remedy

There are a lot of folk remedies that apple cider vinegar has been used for. It can be used to treat such things as sore throats, coughs and sinus relief. These are all the kinds of thing that go hand in hand with the common cold. Most cold relief medicines have added vitamins such as vitamin C and it is thought that this is where apple cider vinegar comes in. The raw form has lots of vitamins, minerals, amino acids and enzymes which can all set about putting the body in the best condition that it can be, in order to fight a cold. It is also said that apple cider vinegar helps to balance a person's acidity level back to normal. It is thought that this acid level is disturbed during a cold infection. If there is a sinus infection apple cider vinegar can help by reducing the amount of mucus that is produced and this in turn helps to stop the pain caused by blocked sinuses. The mucus will turn from a thick green color to a thinner more watery form.

To treat yourself, simply dilute 2 table spoons of the raw vinegar in a large glass of water and drink it throughout the day while you have a cold. Instead of this method you can consume the whole lot and repeat another 2 times a day. You can take the remedy at the start of a cold or for continued protection drink a glass of the diluted apple cider vinegar each day.

You can also sprinkle some apple cider vinegar on your pillow before you sleep. Inhaling the vinegar vapors can help with a persistent cold. For treating a sore throat you can gargle a one to one vinegar to water mixture. Do this every hour making sure you rinse your mouth out with water after each gargle to protect the enamel on your teeth.

Apple cider vinegar for acne

Acne is a skin condition characterized by blocked sebaceous glands. These glands supply important skin conditioning oils to the skin. The glands themselves are situated under the skin surface and a tube leads up to the skin surface so that the oils produced by the gland are released on the skin surface through pores. These oils moisturize the skin and keep it in good condition. This situation works well until the glands become infected with bacteria. These bacteria cause the pore to be blocked and as a result the infected area becomes red and inflamed. It is this inflammation that gives acne its characteristic visual appearance.

Usually the skin has its own helpful bacteria which prevent other bacteria and organisms from infecting the skin and the rest of the body. Unfortunately, changes in the chemical nature of the skin surface can cause these helpful bacteria to die off. This often occurs due to changes within the body due to hormonal control. This is the reason that teenagers are so susceptible to acne. The hormonal changes going on alter the chemical composition of the skin secretions and this reduces the helpful populations of bacteria. This then allows infecting bacteria to get a foot hold. These then can infect the sebaceous gland pores which are often over secreting oils due to the extra hormones as well. This then is the start of the acne condition. In later life the hormonal changes level out; the skin conditions become normal; the helpful bacteria return; the sebaceous glands return to working order; inflammation of the skin reduces and finally the acne disappears.

To deal with acne there are a range of creams and solutions that can be bought from the local chemist shop. These all work on the idea of cleaning the skin and pore areas and killing the bacteria which can infect them. There are also creams which are designed to reduce the inflammation of the skin where the infections occur. These medicines work to a certain extent and people do see positive results in most cases. However, these creams and solutions can also be expensive as well as containing a number of harsh chemical ingredients.

Apple cider vinegar can be used as a more natural remedy for treating acne. It has powerful anti bacterial actions and can therefore work in the same way as some of these creams and solutions from the pharmacy. It can kill the bacterial that cause acne inflammation as well as returning the skin to a more natural acid balance. It also works by removing clogs from the pores of the sebaceous glands as well as dealing with the extra oily secretions from them that add to the conditions causing acne to flare up.

It is relatively easy to use apple cider vinegar to treat acne. To start off with, dilute your apple cider vinegar with water. You should mix 1 part of apple cider vinegar with 4 parts of water. Dip a clean piece of cotton wool into the mixture and then pat it onto the skin. Leave the mixture on the skin for about 10 minutes and then wash it off. Repeat the procedure 2 or 3 times each day until the acne goes away.

Apple cider vinegar can come in various strengths and it is important to dilute it before use on your skin. Although you may get a tingling sensation as you apply it to your skin you certainly shouldn't feel any sensations of burning. If you do get any feelings of burning on your skin, you should check your dilution and if necessary dilute the vinegar some more. Apple cider vinegar can be effective and is a fraction of the cost of the treatments that you can get from a chemist shop. It is also a completely natural product compared to chemical nature of other treatments.

Eczema home remedy

Eczema is a tricky condition to treat. The skin needs to be moisturized and needs to be kept in good condition. There are lots of different creams out there which promise to keep the condition under control. For most people they have success; however, for others they don't seem to work. Sometimes the creams are full of petroleum based products and other artificial ingredients which can cause a bad reaction or make the eczema worse in some people. Apple cider vinegar can help because it contains the vitamin beta carotene which is very good for people with eczema. It also has a lot of potassium which is very good for people suffering from allergies. It is often the case that eczema sufferers often also suffer from allergies and these allergies can trigger the eczema to flare up and vice versa. Amino acids and bioflavonoid in apple cider vinegar can also help by promoting the immune system of people suffering from eczema. Added to this the acetic acid in vinegar helps to deal with bacteria and fungi on the skin surface and this in turn can help to prevent itching and dryness of the skin. These properties of apple cider vinegar are very important for eczema sufferers. To get relief from itching you should try a solution made up of half and half of water and apple cider vinegar. Apply this to the affected area and the itching should go away pretty quickly.

Apple cider vinegar as a skin toner

You can make an excellent skin toner using apple cider vinegar. This fantastic toner is free from man made chemicals and on top of this is far cheaper than buying a skin toner from a chemist shop or a supermarket. Apple cider vinegar has the benefit of having lots of natural alpha hydroxyl acid ions it. These, together with amino acids in the vinegar, tone the skin by removing dead skin cells, correcting the acid balance of the skin and stimulating blood flow. Alpha hydroxyl acids are well known in the cosmetics industry where they are used to try and reduce aging and wrinkles in the skin. The main ingredient in apple cider vinegar is acetic acid and this too stimulates the flow of blood in the small blood vessels under the skin. This then helps to give skin a soft glow which is pleasing to the eye.

The toner is simply made by combining one part apple cider vinegar with one part distilled water in a jug and then mixing it well. Use the toner by dipping a cotton ball into the mixture and then gently applying to the skin. Test a small area of skin before using it extensively, just in case your skin reacts against it.

You can improve the basic toner by mixing green tea with it. Make some green tea in the usual way using a tea bag with boiling water and let it brew for about 15 minutes and then leave to cool. Once this is done remove the tea bag and add the green tea liquor to the toner so that there are equal amounts of green tea, water and vinegar in it. The green tea is good for the skin because it contains lots of valuable antioxidants. This toner can help to stop skin wrinkles and even dark circles under the eyes. Be careful not to get the toner in the eyes themselves as it will sting.

You can also add chamomile flowers to the green tea while it is brewing. This then makes an herbal infusion. Strain off the chamomile flowers and then add a teaspoon each of aloe vera and rose water. This makes a very gentle skin toner. You need to keep this refrigerated and make sure that you use it up within a month.

Osteoporosis

This is a bone disease which is associated with older people especially women. It is a crippling condition which can cause a huge amount of pain. It is caused by the bones losing calcium salts. Calcium salts are important for keeping bones strong because the salts are deposited in the bone structure where they become as hard as stone. Together with the organic materials in bone they form a very strong structure which could be considered to be a bit like reinforced concrete. Bones can therefore survive impacts and bending forces without getting broken. Obviously everybody knows of people who have broken bones in their body but these breaks in healthy people will be due to the extreme forces that you get in an accident of some kind. Bones won't break during normal use. In the case of osteoporosis the bones start to lose their calcium content which makes them a lot weaker. This weakness causes the stooping image of older people where the backbone becomes bent due to the lack of calcium salts in its structure.

In women one of the main causes of bone loss is attributed to the changing nature of hormone levels during the menopause. In the early stages of the menopause things can be corrected by the use of hormone replacement therapy but this is not suitable for everybody. Later in life there are calcium building drugs that doctors can prescribe. These drugs are designed to get the bones to hang onto their calcium rather than losing it. In addition to this people with osteoporosis are also given calcium tablets to increase their dietary consumption of this important mineral.

Apple cider vinegar is reckoned to help with osteoporosis and a lot of people swear by its use. This might seem a bit strange to some people as they may recollect that acids will remove minerals from bones if they are soaked in it. Well, this is part of 101 Biology I guess! However, it is not the direct action of vinegar acid on bones that we should be concerned with. Rather, it is the action of the acetic acid in apple cider vinegar on the digestive system.

The acid in vinegar has been shown to help in the absorption of minerals from the food that we eat. These minerals will of course include calcium. As a result drinking vinegar with or before meals could help your body to absorb calcium from the food that you eat. You still have to make sure that you eat food that is rich in calcium though.

Adding apple cider vinegar to the diet could therefore be useful for women who are having problems getting enough calcium from their diet to maintain the levels in their bones. This is doubly important for people who have lactose intolerance and can't consume dairy products. Dairy products are very rich in calcium and can make up a considerable amount of the calcium that we consume during our normal diets. People with lactose intolerance have to look elsewhere for their calcium. Although leafy vegetables with a dark green color often contain lots of calcium they may also contain other substances which tend to stop the calcium being absorbed from the gut. Apple cider vinegar can therefore be used to fight against these substances and improve calcium absorption from the digestive system.

Arthritis

Apple cider vinegar is folk cure for the joint condition called arthritis. There isn't really any scientific evidence that can be produced to support the action of vinegar on this condition. On the other hand, there isn't really a great understanding of how to cure or treat arthritis, even using modern medicines. Most drugs prescribed for the condition can to a certain extent control the pain produced by arthritis but they certainly can't cure it. People with the condition are often prepared to try all sorts of methods to treat it and get relief. As a result, if you are looking for something else to try then Apple cider vinegar could be worth a go.

The popular belief of apple cider vinegar as a treatment for arthritis began with a nurse called Margaret Hills. She suffered from arthritis when she was just under 40 years old and did a lot of research into the best treatments for the condition. She tried apple cider vinegar and found that the arthritis was relieved and later didn't suffer from the condition any more. She had found the idea of the treatment by following the advice of a Dr Jarvis.

Dr Jarvis had proposed that arthritis was caused by the deposition of calcium salts in the joints. He reckoned that the high potassium content and other nutrients in raw apple cider vinegar was responsible for the removal of these calcium salts and the regeneration of new tissue in the damaged joints. This in turn gave relief from the pain and disability caused by the arthritis. He stressed the importance of using raw vinegar rather than the treated and pasteurized form found in many health food shops. This treated form of apple cider vinegar lacks a lot of the nutrients and active ingredients found in the raw form.

Margaret Hill was so impressed with way that apple cider vinegar had worked for her that she set up a clinic to treat others. She followed the recommendations of Dr Jarvis in the use of a mixture of 1 table spoon of apple cider vinegar and 1 tablespoon of honey mixed in a glass of warm water to be consumed three times a day. People started with 1 treatment per day and gradually worked up to the full 3 a day method.

Apple cider vinegar and gout

Gout is an old fashioned kind of ailment which appears to be coming back. It was said to be due to rich living! It is caused by a build up of uric acid in the body. This then causes uric acid crystals to appear in joints and this is what causes the pain associated with gout. This is thought to be related to diet. In past such things as drinking too much port was thought to be to blame.

Apple cider vinegar has always been a favorite folk remedy for gout. It is important once again to use the raw unpasteurized version of the vinegar because it will contain all of the active ingredients such as amino acids and proteins which can be destroyed by heating.

You should make a mixture of 2 tablespoons of vinegar with water in a large glass. Drink this mixture twice a day. It is thought that the apple cider vinegar works by stabilizing the acid levels within your blood and that this then helps to remove the uric acid from the joints where it has collected causing the gout. You can also apply the mixture to skin where the gout condition is giving the pain. This will then help to reduce any inflammation and ease the pain. You can also make a warm soak to ease the condition. Use one part vinegar to 6 part warm water and soak the affected area in it for about half an hour.

As with all joint problems involving arthritis symptoms you should consult a health professional if the condition doesn't get better.

Apple cider vinegar for hair

Apple cider vinegar can be used to give your hair some life. Use a rinse of apple cider vinegar to remove the build up of hair styling materials and to give a real bounce and shine to your hair. The acetic acid in vinegar can get rid of excess conditioning products and strengthen your hair at the same time. Once used you are left with soft and shining hair that will make you feel good all over.

In addition to this the apple cider vinegar will also even out the acid and alkaline balance of your hair allowing it to grow strong and healthy. It has antibacterial properties and will also cure your dandruff. I have been using it for my dandruff for a long time now. Before this, I was buying expensive Chinese herbal products to do the same job but without the same success. Don't use apple cider vinegar with colored hair as it can remove the color.

To make the apple cider rinse, mix a third of a cup of the vinegar with two pints of distilled or purified water and put it into a suitable bottle. Once in the shower, shampoo your hair as normal and then rinse out the lather well. Next put the apple cider rinse on your hair and leave it in for a few seconds to work. After this rinse your hair one again. Use cold water as this will seal the hair and produce a far better shine. Only use your rinse once a week to maintain the condition of your hair. After using the rinse you don't have to use a normal conditioner.

Everybody's hair is different so keep a check on how your hair reacts to the vinegar and change your use of it according to the results that you get. The next thing to do is to dry your hair with a towel. If you smell vinegar after rinsing out with cold water you shouldn't worry because any residual smell will go once you have dried your hair.

You can also add a few drops of fragrance in the form of essential oils to make sure the vinegar isn't noticed at all. You could use lavender, rosemary. Lemon, rose or vanilla for this purpose. I usually use vanilla and I find that with this there is no smell of vinegar left at all.

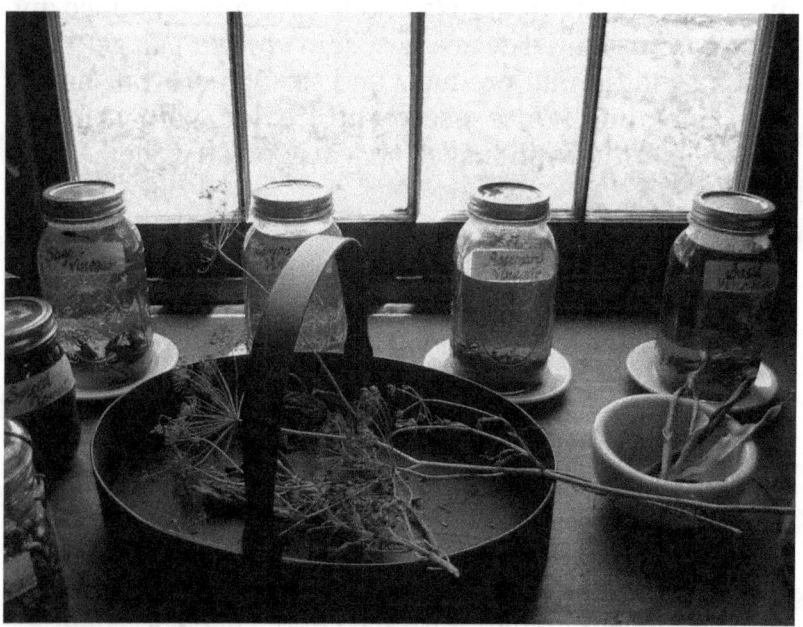

You can also make a simple herbal style apple cider vinegar rinse by first adding the herbs to a cup of boiling water and letting the mixture infuse for about 2 hours. Use about 3 table spoons of the herbs, or as much as you need. Once the infusion is cool add a cup of the apple cider vinegar and mix it in well. You can use this infused version in the same way as the ordinary apple cider vinegar rinse. The herbs that you use are a personal choice but rosemary is good for brown hair, chamomile with blond hair. Marigold is good for dry hair, lavender with oily hair and burdock for hair growth.

Apple cider vinegar in cooking

Apple cider vinegar has many uses in cooking. It can be both a tasty ingredient as well as an active agent in preservation and keeping foods free from moulds. Just about all condiments that we have on our table such as tomato and brown sauces have vinegar as a main ingredient. Apple cider vinegar can be substituted for any other types of vinegar in these condiments. As well as enhancing flavours in many dishes it can also be used to make meat tenderer before it is cooked. In the case of baking bread, apple cider vinegar can be used to make the crust of home baked bread have a shinier glaze.

Here are some more specific ways that you can use apple cider vinegar in your general cooking.

With fruits and vegetables you can use apple cider vinegar in their preparation. It can be used to help remove any insects and other bugs as well as any chemicals which may have been sprayed on them. Use a solution made up of 1 tablespoon of apple cider vinegar in 5 litres of water and allow the fruits and vegetables to soak in it a while. After soaking rinse them in water to remove any residues. To get rid of bacteria on the fruit and vegetables increase the concentration of the soaking solution to 2 tablespoons of apple cider vinegar in 5 litres of water and use the same process.

Apple cider vinegar can be used to stop fruits and vegetables from going brown on the cut edges. This is especially true for fruits such as apples and pears and potatoes. The browning is caused by phenols and other substances becoming oxidised when they are exposed to the air. Use a soaking solution of 1 tablespoon of apple cider vinegar in 5 litres of water. These oxidising reactions can be reduced further by keeping the soaking fruits and vegetables cool in the refrigerator or by adding ice or both. Using this method will also help to preserve the vitamin C content of your vegetables as it is very susceptible to oxidation as well.

There are also advantages of using apple cider vinegar in the cooking process with vegetables. If you use a tablespoon of apple cider vinegar in the water used to steam vegetables you will find that bright colours are less likely to be lost. Dried beans always have a problem of causing gas when being eaten. The amount of gas can be reduced by adding apple cider vinegar to the water that they are pre-soaked in and also to the water that is used to cook them in. The smell that comes from cabbage as it is cooked can be reduced by adding some vinegar to the water that it is cooked in.

In terms of fruit, adding a teaspoon of vinegar as it is cooking will help to make it taste better. This works well when cooking apples for pies and so on. Adding apple cider vinegar to fruit gelatine will help to keep it nice and firm.

You can also use the preservative nature of apple cider vinegar to keep any left over items such as ginger and garlic, if they have already been cut up. Usually these would be wasted if not used straight away. However, they can be stored by covering them with apple cider vinegar in a glass jar and placing them in the refrigerator until they are next needed.

In the case of eggs, you can use apple cider vinegar when cooking them. When you are boiling eggs, add a tablespoon or 2 to the water. This will stop the white part of the eggs leaking from any cracks in the egg shell. Likewise, you can help to maintain the shape of poached eggs by adding 1 or 2 tablespoons to the boiling water in the pan. At Easter time apple cider vinegar can be used together with hot water and food colouring. When the eggs are added to the colouring it should help to both prevent the colours streaking and make the colours nice and bright.

Marinating meat is an important way of adding flavour. Vinegar is often a part of the marinade used with meats. The longer that the meat is soaked in the marinade then the more flavour that is absorbed by it. Apple cider vinegar also has the benefit of killing bacteria on the meat and making it tenderer. For a good marinade use a quarter of a cup of apple cider vinegar and then add herbs and spices to get different flavours. Rub the marinade over the meat and allow it to soak into the surfaces. If the meat is very tough then it is best to leave it soaking in the marinade over night in the refrigerator. .

Barbeque sauces can also be made by using apple cider vinegar as the base. Once again add herbs and spices to emphasise different flavours. This sauce will then add extra flavour as well as tenderizing the meat. When used on wild meat, apple cider vinegar will help by emphasizing the game flavours involved. It is best to soak the wild meat in the vinegar before cooking it.

With boiled meats such as ham, putting a tablespoon of apple cider vinegar in the water used for cooking it will help the flavour to come out as well as making it tender and producing a better texture. If salt is included in the meat as is the case with gammon joints adding apple cider vinegar will help to reduce the salty taste of the meat.

Apple cider vinegar can also be used with fish. When preparing fish, you will find that rubbing the fish with apple cider vinegar will help you in removing the scales. Once again apple cider vinegar can be used to bring out the natural flavour of the fish and also tenderize it. Simply soak the fish in apple cider vinegar before you cook it. Apple cider vinegar can also improve the taste of canned fish such as tuna or salmon.

In baking bread you will find that adding a tablespoon of apple cider vinegar will help the bread to rise. Simply add a tablespoon less of water and then substitute the apple cider vinegar in its place. As the baking time nears its end you should brush the top of the baking bread with apple cider vinegar in order to increase the shiny glaze produced. Once you have brushed the surface replace the bread back in the oven for a few minutes longer to complete the baking.

You can bake fluffier meringues by beating the egg whites with apple cider vinegar. When baking pies using flaky pastry add a tablespoon of apple cider vinegar to the pastry recipe and you will find that the pie crust produced will be superior to the normal kind that you make. In addition to this adding apple cider vinegar to dessert pie contents will increase the flavour produced and also reduce the overall sweetness of the pie.

There are a number of other instances when apple cider vinegar can be used to enhance the results of cooking food. Here are some extra little tricks which can help you in the kitchen:

In the case of pasta, adding a tablespoon of the vinegar to the water used for cooking it instead of salt will not only reduce the salt content but will also help to prevent the pasta sticking.

Rice can also be made to be fluffier by adding a teaspoon of apple cider vinegar when you cook it.

Preserve olives and pimento peppers by covering them with apple cider vinegar and keeping them in the refrigerator. This is especially the case if you have olives that have come out of a jar with a limited shelf life.

Cheese often has a problem of becoming both dried out a covered with mould when stored in the refrigerator for any length of time. You can prevent both of these conditions by covering the cheese with a cloth that has been soaked in apple cider vinegar. Keep the cheese in this way in an air tight container in your refrigerator.

We often put lemon on fried foods such as fish but you can equally use apple cider vinegar instead to get a variation in flavour.

Apple cider vinegar recipes

Homemade sour cream

Ingredients

1 cup cottage cheese
¼ cup skimmed milk
1 tsp apple cider vinegar

Method

Blend together the cottage cheese, skimmed milk and apple cider vinegar until you have a nice creamy mixture.

Homemade Buttermilk

Ingredients

1 tbsp apple cider vinegar
1 cup milk

Method

Add the apple cider vinegar to the milk and then leave it to stand for 5 minutes or so. After this time it should have thickened into a nice buttermilk.

Apple cider vinegar French dressing

Ingredients

1 ½ tsp Dijon mustard
1 tsp sugar
¼ tsp salt
¼ tsp freshly ground black pepper
1/3 cup apple cider vinegar
1 tbsp chopped flat leaf parsley
2/3 cup extra virgin olive oil

Method

Put the Dijon mustard, sugar, pepper, vinegar and chopped parsley into a mixing bowl and then whisk them together.

Whisk the mixture consistently as you slowly add the olive oil. Keep whisking until the mixture becomes thickened.

Add more salt and pepper to taste. You can use it as soon as it is ready or store it in the refrigerator for use later. You can keep the French dressing in the refrigerator for about 2 days. Make sure that you return it to room temperature before you use it.

Cos lettuce hearts with an apple cider vinaigrette

Ingredients

1 ¼ cups extra virgin olive oil
1/3 cup apple cider vinegar
3 tbsp apple juice concentrate
2 tbsp finely chopped red onion
1 tsp salt
½ tsp ground nutmeg
½ tsp ground ginger
¼ tsp freshly ground black pepper
1 cup thinly sliced red onion
2 large apples
5 hearts of Cos lettuce
¾ cup pecans coarsely chopped and toasted

Method

Make the salad dressing by first putting the olive oil, apple cider vinegar, apple juice, chopped red onion, salt, nutmeg, ginger and black pepper into a small bowl. Whisk together until the ingredients are well blended together. You can make this the day before and store in the refrigerator for use the next day. Make sure you whisk it again after removing it from the refrigerator.

Put the sliced red onion into a large bowl and cover it with cold water. Leave the onion to soak for about half an hour. Meanwhile core and peel the apples and then dice into ¼ inch pieces.

After 30 minutes drain the water from the onions. Put a 1/3 cup of the salad dressing into a medium bowl and then add the diced apple. Toss the mixture until the diced apple is well coated.

Trim and then cut the Cos lettuce hearts along their length until each is made up of 3 wedge shapes. Fan out the Cos lettuce wedges on a large serving plate and then top it off with the sliced red onion. Drizzle the salad with the dressing and then finish it off by sprinkling with the chopped pecan nuts.

Baked chicken in an apple cider vinegar marinade

Ingredients

2 cups apple cider vinegar
1 cup extra virgin olive oil
1 egg
3 tsp salt
1 tsp chicken seasoning
8 boneless chicken thighs with skin

Method

Lightly beat the egg and then place it into a large bowl. Mix in the apple cider vinegar, olive oil, salt and chicken seasoning. Once it is mixed well add the chicken thighs and make sure that they are covered by the mixture. Place the bowl in the refrigerator and leave the chicken to marinate for an hour.

Put the chicken thighs in a baking dish and cover them with about a quarter of the marinade. Place the dish into a preheated oven set to 180C and bake for about 30 minutes.

After 30 minutes remove the dish from the oven and drain off the excess marinade. Place the dish back into the oven and cook for a further 15 minutes or until the chicken skin becomes crisp. Make sure that the chicken meat is no longer pink and that the juices from the meat are clear.

Spinach Salad with apple cider vinegar and Bacon

Ingredients

1 cup extra virgin olive oil
1 tsp powdered sugar
¼ cup apple cider vinegar
1 tbsp fresh lemon juice
1 ½ tsp dry mustard
1 ½ tsp paprika
½ tsp ground ginger
½ lb bacon
12 oz baby spinach leaves
2 apples
1 medium red onion
1 ripe avocado
Salt and pepper seasoning

Method

Put the powdered sugar, apple cider vinegar, lemon juice, mustard, paprika and ginger into a bowl and whisk until the ingredients are well blended. Add salt and pepper seasoning to taste. Keep this dressing for use later.

Chop the slices of bacon and then cook them in a frying pan on a medium heat until the pieces become nice and crisp and browned. Once they are cooked drain off any excess fat and move the bacon pieces onto paper towel to drain.

Core the apples and then cut them into halves and thinly slice them. Thinly slice the red onion. Halve the avocado and remove the stone from it. Peel the avocado halves and then chop them into cubes. Put the baby spinach leaves, apple slices, red onion slices, avocado cubes and bacon bits into a large bowl and gently mix to combine the ingredients.

Toss the salad in the large bowl with enough of the salad dressing to coat all of the ingredients.

Slow cooked chicken stew with apple cider vinegar

Ingredients

4 potatoes
4 carrots
1 red onion
1 celery rib
1 tsp salt
¾ tsp dried thyme
½ tsp pepper
¼ tsp caraway seeds
2 lbs boneless and skinless chicken breast
2 tbsp extra virgin olive oil
1 tart apple
1 ¼ cups apple cider
1 tbsp apple cider vinegar

1 bay leaf
Chopped fresh parsley

Method

Peel and cut the potatoes into cubes. Chop the carrots into slices that are about ¼ inch in thickness. Halve the red onion and cut it into thin slices. Thinly slice the celery rib. Peel and core the apple and then cut it into cubes. Dice the chicken breast into mouth sized cubes.

Layer the potatoes, carrots, celery and onion in the bottom of a slow cooker. Mix together the salt, thyme, pepper and caraway seeds in a small bowl. Sprinkle about half of this seasoning over the vegetables in the slow cooker.

Fry the chicken cubes in the olive oil over a medium heat until they are evenly browned. Put the cooked chicken into the slow cooker in a layer over the vegetables. Sprinkle the apple cubes over the chicken.

Mix the apple cider and the apple cider vinegar and then pour it over the chicken and apple in the slow cooker. Next sprinkle the remaining seasoning mixture on the top of everything. Finally place the bay leaf on the top.

Cover with the slow cooker lid and set to cook for about 5 or 6 hours until both the vegetables and chicken are well cooked.

On serving, remove the bay leaf and garnish with the chopped parsley.

Apple cider vinegar chicken

Ingredients

1 tbsp extra virgin olive oil
1 onion
4 lbs chicken
29 oz can of tomato sauce
3 ½ cups apple cider vinegar
Salt
Pepper
1 pinch garlic powder
Fresh basil

Method

Thinly slice the onion and cut the chicken into bite sized pieces. Place the onion into a large frying pan and cook in the olive oil until it becomes translucent. At this point add the chicken pieces to the pan and continue to cook until the chicken is evenly browned.

Once the chicken is brown add the tomato sauce to the pan followed by the apple cider vinegar. Season with salt and pepper and add the garlic powder. Mix this all together in the pan and then heat until the mixture starts to boil. Reduce the heat and then continue to simmer for about 30 minutes. After this time check that the chicken is tender and well cooked. Serve with a fresh basil garnish.

Spinach and apple cider vinegar salad

Ingredients

2 tbsp apple cider vinegar
2 tbsp extra virgin olive oil
¼ tsp salt
¼ tsp sugar
1 cup apples
¼ cup sweet onion
¼ cup raisins
2 cups of roughly torn spinach
2 cups of roughly torn Cos lettuce

Method

Core the apple and then dice it including the skin. Chop the sweet onion.

Put the apple cider vinegar, olive oil, salt and sugar into a bowl and mix it well. Add the diced apple, chopped onion and the raisins. Stir the mixture until the apple pieces are well coated in the mixture. Cover the salad dressing and leave it to stand for about 30 minutes.

Combine the spinach and Cos lettuce pieces in a large serving bowl and then add the salad dressing made earlier. Toss the salad so that it combines evenly with the dressing.

Cheddar and apple salad with apple cider vinegar

Ingredients

10 cups roughly torn mixed salad greens
1 cup chopped red apple
1 cup cubed cheddar cheese
1 cup toasted chopped walnuts
2/3 cup honey
2 tbsp apple cider vinegar
1 tsp celery seed
1 tsp ground mustard
1 tsp paprika
1 tsp lemon juice
1 tsp grated onion
¼ tsp salt
1 cup extra virgin olive oil

Method

Put the honey, apple cider vinegar, celery seeds, mustard, paprika, lemon juice, onion and salt into a blender. During the blending process slowly add the olive oil. Blend the mixture until a smooth salad dressing is formed.

Put the salad greens, apple, cheddar cheese and chopped walnuts into a large salad bowl and gently combine them together. Toss the salad greens with the salad dressing and serve.

Apple, Beet and Avocado Salad

Ingredients

3 beetroot
¼ cup water
4 cups mixed salad greens
1 onion
1 apple
½ avocado
½ cup toasted chopped walnuts
¾ cup apple cider
2/3 cup apple cider vinegar
½ cup extra virgin olive oil
½ tsp salt
½ tsp freshly ground black pepper
1 tsp prepared mustard
¼ tsp celery seed

Method

Wash the beetroot and put them into a baking dish. Add the water to the dish and cover with a lid. Bake the beetroot in a preheated oven set to 200C for about an hour or until the beetroot are tender. Once they are cooked remove them from the oven and leave them to cool.

Slice the onion into thin rings. Core and peel the apple and then thinly slice it. Halve the avocado to remove the stone and then peel and slice it.

Put the apple cider, apple cider vinegar, olive oil, salt, pepper, mustard and celery seeds into a medium sized bowl and whisk to combine the ingredients to form a vinaigrette.

Once the beetroots are cool, peel and slice them. Add these to the vinaigrette and then place the bowl into the refrigerator. Leave the mixture in the refrigerator for about an hour so that the flavours mix and develop.

Combine the avocado, mixed greens and onion slices in a large salad bowl and then add the beetroot and vinaigrette mixture. Toss the salad with the vinaigrette and then sprinkle with the nuts.

Apple cider vinegar BBQ Sauce

Ingredients

2 cups tomato ketchup
1 cup water
½ cup apple cider vinegar
5 tbsp light brown sugar
5 tbsp sugar
½ tbsp fresh ground black pepper
½ tbsp onion powder
½ tbsp ground mustard
1 tbsp lemon juice
1 tbsp Worcestershire sauce

Method

Place all of the ingredients into a medium sized saucepan. Heat the mixture until it gets to boiling point and then reduce the heat until it is simmering. Keep the saucepan uncovered and continue to simmer, while stirring often, for about an hour and a quarter. Use this BBQ sauce with both fish and meat dishes.

Green tomato chutney

Ingredients

1 lemon
1 clove garlic
5 cups of chopped firm green tomatoes
2 ¼ cups brown sugar
1 ½ cups seeded raisins
¾ cup chopped fresh ginger root
1 ½ tsp cayenne pepper
2 cups apple cider vinegar
2 red peppers

Method

Remove the seeds from the lemon and then chop it up. Remove the skin from the garlic clove and then chop this too. Remove the seeds from the red peppers and chop them.

Add all of the ingredients to a large saucepan and heat until the mixture is boiling. Reduce the heat to a simmer and continue to cook until everything is nice and tender. Put the cooked chutney into sterile jars and seal them.

Grilled apple cider vinegar marinated pork chops

Ingredients

6 shoulder pork chops
6 oz apple juice concentrate
1/3 cup apple jelly

¼ cup extra virgin olive oil
3 tbsp apple cider vinegar
2 tbsp Worcestershire sauce
2 tbsp Dijon style mustard
2 tsp dried rosemary
1 tsp dried sage
2 tsp salt
1 tsp ground black pepper

Method

Put the apple juice, apple jelly, olive oil, Worcestershire sauce, mustard, rosemary, sage, salt and pepper into a blender and process them to make the marinade.

Place the pork chops in a shallow dish and then coat them with the marinade. Cover the dish and then put it into the refrigerator so that the chops can marinate over night.

Remove the chops from the marinade and then cook on a preheated BBQ or grill for about 8 or 9 minutes on each side. Make sure that the chops are cooked through and then serve.

Ginger chutney

Ingredients

3 cups apple cider vinegar
4 cups brown sugar
4 to 5 lbs tart apples
4 lemons with rinds
2 med. sized onions
5 large garlic cloves
½ cup peeled and finely chopped fresh ginger

1 ½ cups dark raisins
1 tsp cayenne pepper

Method

Peel core and then dice the apples. Chop the whole of the lemon including the rind and then remove the seeds. Chop the onions and then chop the garlic cloves.

Put the apple cider vinegar and sugar into a large saucepan and heat until it begins to simmer. Next stir in the diced apples and continue to heat until it starts to simmer once again. Stir in the lemon pieces, chopped onions, garlic, cloves, ginger, raisins and cayenne pepper. Cook the mixture by simmering it gently for about 30 minutes. Make sure that you stir the pot every now and then.

Once cooking is complete transfer the ginger chutney into sterilised glass jars and seal them up. You should keep the chutney in the refrigerator and use within about 5 weeks.

Apple cider vinegar and Swiss cheese salad

Ingredients

Mixed salad greens
1 large sweet apple
1 tbsp lemon juice
½ cup sliced red onion
4 oz Swiss cheese
½ cup extra virgin olive oil
6 tbsp apple cider vinegar

2 tbsp sugar
4 tsp Dijon mustard
1/3 cup walnut pieces

Method

Tear the mixed salad greens into bite sized pieces until you have about 6 cups. Core the apple and then cut it into quarters and then slices. Cut the Swiss cheese into cubes of about a half inch in size.

Put the torn salad greens into a large salad bowl. In another smaller bowl put the apple and lemon juices. Stir these to coat the apple and leave for a while for the lemon to be absorbed. Drain off the excess lemon juice and then add the apple to the large bowl with the salad greens. Next add the red onion slices and the cheese cubes.

Put the olive oil, apple cider vinegar, sugar and mustard into a jar with a secure lid and shake to mix in order to make the salad dressing.

Drizzle the salad dressing over the salad in the large bowl and toss it so that the greens become coated with the dressing. Sprinkle the walnut pieces over the salad and serve.

Beef and apple cider vinegar stew

Ingredients

4 ½ tbsp plain flour
3 tsp salt
1 ½ tsp freshly ground pepper
½ tsp thyme

3 lb stewing steak
4 ½ tbsp extra virgin olive oil
3 cups apple cider
¾ cup water
3 tbsp apple cider vinegar
6 carrots
5 potatoes
3 onions
4 celery sticks
2 apples
Sliced mushrooms

Method

Mix the flour, salt and pepper and thyme in a large bowl. Cut the stewing steak into cubes and then shake the meat in the flour mixture so that the cubes of meat become coated.

Add the coated meat to a large frying pan with the olive oil and then cook on a medium heat until the meat becomes browned.

Put the cider, water and vinegar into a large saucepan and then add the partly cooked meat. Heat the mixture until boiling and then reduce the heat until it is simmering. Continue to cook for about 2 hours until the meat is nice and tender.

Chop the celery sticks and apple. Quarter the carrots and the potatoes and then add them all to the saucepan together with the onions, celery, apples and as many mushrooms as you desire. Continue to cook until the vegetables are nice and tender.

Penne Pasta with lima beans in an apple cider vinaigrette

Ingredients

1 lb penne rigate pasta
¾ cup safflower oil
2 cups cooked fresh corn kernels
2 cups cooked fresh lima beans
2 medium sized tomatoes
8 thinly sliced green onions
6 strips thick sliced bacon
1/3 cup chopped fresh parsley
3 tbsp apple cider vinegar
2 tbsp freshly squeezed lemon juice
1 tsp granulated sugar
Salt
Freshly ground black pepper
Paprika

Method

Peel the tomatoes, remove the seeds and then chop them.

Fry the bacon until it is nice and crisp. Leave to cool on paper towel and then crumble it up.

Put the pasta into 8 pints of boiling salted water and cook until it is al dente. Drain the pasta and then toss it with ¼ cup of safflower oil in a large bowl. Once the pasta is coated leave it to cool.

Next add the cooked corn and lima beans followed by the chopped tomatoes and onion. Add about ¾ of the crumbled bacon and the parsley. Mix the ingredients with the pasta until they are well combined.

To make the vinaigrette mix ½ cup of safflower oil with the apple cider vinegar, lemon juice, sugar, salt, pepper and paprika seasoning. Pour the vinaigrette over the pasta and make sure that it is mixed in well. Sprinkle on the remaining crumbled bacon and serve.

Sausage and apple cider vinegar bake

Ingredients

1 lb Polish sausage
3 tbsp butter
½ head Savoy cabbage
1/3 cup water
2 green apples
¼ cup brown sugar
¼ cup apple cider vinegar
1 tsp salt
1 ½ tsp dry English mustard
1/8 tsp pepper

Method

Shred the Savoy cabbage. Core and chop one of the apples and then core and slice the remaining one.

Slice the sausage and then fry it in a pan until it is browned. Drain off any excess fat and then add the onions and 2 tbsp of butter and cook until they are golden brown.

Add the shredded cabbage and the water and then cook for about another 10 minutes until the cabbage is nice and tender. Drain off any excess liquid and then mix in the chopped apple.

Pour the mixture into a casserole dish and then layer the apple slices on the top.

Mix the sugar, apple cider vinegar, salt, mustard and pepper together and then stir in a tablespoon of melted butter. Pour this mixture over the layer of apples in the casserole dish and then cover with the casserole lid.

Bake in a preheated oven set to 190C for around 40 minutes and then serve while nice and hot.

Spicy apple relish with apple cider vinegar

Ingredients

1 cup sugar
1 tbsp prepared mustard
1/3 cup apple cider vinegar
2/3 cup water
4 whole allspice
1 stick cinnamon
1 piece crystallized ginger
4 green apples
½ cup seedless raisins
½ cup chopped walnuts

Method

Core and then chop the apples into reasonably sized pieces.

Mix the sugar and mustard together in a large saucepan. Once they are well blended stir in the water and the apple cider vinegar. Next throw in the cinnamon, ginger and the allspice. Bring the mixture to the boil and then reduce the heat to a simmer. Continue to simmer on a low heat for about 12 minutes. At this point take out the spices and discard them.

Add the chopped apples to the pan and return to a gentle simmer. Stir the mixture to make sure that the apple pieces cook evenly, but don't overcook them. Once the apple is tender add the raisins and chopped walnuts and then take away from the heat. Pour the relish into suitable jars and then chill in the refrigerator before using.

Onions in a spicy apple cider vinegar sauce

Ingredients

4 large onions
3 tbsp apple jelly
2 tbsp hot mustard
1 tbsp grated ginger root
1 tbsp apple cider vinegar
1 tbsp cornstarch
1 cup apple cider

Method

Peel the onions and then cut them into halves. Place the onions into a microwave safe dish and then add about an inch of water around them. Place a lid on the dish and then cook in the microwave on full power for about 20 minutes. Make sure that the onions are tender and if not cook for a little while longer.

Put the apple jelly, mustard, ginger, apple cider vinegar and corn starch into a saucepan. Whisk these ingredients until they are blended together. Next add the apple cider and stir to combine with the other ingredients. Cook over a medium heat while stirring until the sauce becomes thick and it begins to boil.

Drain the water from the cooked onions and then serve them together with the apple cider vinegar sauce. This is a nice accompaniment to go with roasted meats such as ham, pork, chicken and turkey.

Red cabbage with apple cider vinegar

Ingredients

3 medium onions
3 tbsp butter
3 large apples
1 small red cabbage
¼ cup apple cider vinegar
2/3 cup water
1 tsp salt
1 tbsp sugar
½ tsp nutmeg

Method

Chop the onions and apples and then shred the red cabbage.

Cook the onions in the butter in a sauce pan on a medium heat. Once they are a golden brown colour add the apple, red cabbage, apple cider vinegar, water, salt, sugar and nutmeg. Put the lid on the saucepan and then gently cook for about 30 minutes. Make sure that the red cabbage is tender before serving.

Piquant chicken and apple cider vinegar

Ingredients

2 chicken breasts
1 tbsp extra virgin olive oil
1 apple
1 onion
2 tbsp apple cider vinegar
¼ tsp paprika
1/8 tsp cinnamon powder
1/8 tsp ground ginger
Pinch of pepper

Method

Cut the apple into wedges and chop up the onion.

Dice the chicken breasts and then cook in a large saucepan pan in the olive oil until it is browned nicely and no longer pink.

Next add the apple, onion, apple cider vinegar, paprika, cinnamon, ginger and pepper. Also add a little water so that the chicken doesn't stick to the pan.

Cook on a medium heat until boiling and then put the lid on the saucepan, reduce the heat and simmer for about 20 minutes. Serve with boiled rice for a tasty low calorie meal.

Apple bread

Ingredients

3 cups plain flour
1 ½ tsp baking soda
1 1/3 tsp salt
1 ½ tsp cinnamon
¾ tsp nutmeg
½ tsp allspice
¼ tsp ground cloves
¾ cup shortening
1 1/8 cup brown sugar
3 eggs
1 ½ tsp vanilla
1 ½ cup grated apples
3 tbsp apple cider vinegar
½ cup water
¾ cup chopped walnuts

Method

Sift the flour into a medium bowl and then add the baking soda, salt, cinnamon, nutmeg, allspice and cloves. Mix until the ingredients are well combined.

Cream together the shortening with the sugar in another bowl using a whisk. Next add the eggs one at a time while beating with the whisk. Add the vanilla and stir to mix in.

Stir in the flour mixture slowly while adding the apples, apple cider vinegar and water. Make sure the ingredients are well combines and the finally stir in the chopped walnuts.

Pour the batter into a greased bread pan and then bake in a preheated oven set to 200C for about an hour or so until cooked to your liking. Leave the bread to cool on a wire rack before serving.

Apple cider vinegar and honey fruit dressing

Ingredients

1/3 cup fructose syrup
¼ tsp dry mustard
½ tsp paprika
¼ tsp coarse salt
½ cup apple sauce
¼ cup honey
3 tbsp lemon juice
1 tbsp apple cider vinegar
¼ tsp grated lemon peel
½ cup canola oil

Method

Put the fructose, mustard, paprika, salt, apple sauce, honey, lemon juice, apple cider vinegar and lemon peel in a medium sized bowl. Mix these ingredients to combine them well.

Slowly add the canola oil as you beat the mixture with a whisk. Make sure that the mixture is beaten well. Put the fruit dressing in the refrigerator for about an hour and then beat well, once again, before serving. This dressing goes very well with fruit. Simply pour the dressing over the fruit and enjoy.

Health risks of apple cider vinegar

The health risks of taking small amounts of apple cider every now and then would seem to be very small. However, taking apple cider vinegar on a regular basis over a longer period of time or taking bigger amounts of it could have some risk. You should always consult your doctor if you are considering taking apple cider vinegar for a persistent or more serious ailment. You should think about the impact of the following things before using apple cider vinegar on a more long term basis.

Apple cider vinegar contains the acid known as acetic acid. This acid can be quite harsh in its raw form and as a result you should always dilute it with water before drinking it. The strength of the acid in the raw form can definitely damage the enamel on teeth and possibly the skin tissue of the throat, mouth and esophagus. Damage to teeth is generally associated with sipping the vinegar. The longer it is in contact with the teeth the greater the effect. Therefore swallowing it straight away is preferable. In addition to this using water as a mouth wash after talking vinegar will allow the teeth to re-calcify themselves. Certainly you shouldn't brush your teeth directly after sipping the vinegar as the brushing will remove any attacked enamel before it has had a chance to re-calcify.

The use of apple cider vinegar over long periods of time could possibly lead to low potassium levels in the body and lower bone density. As a result people with lower potassium levels or suffering from osteoporosis need to discuss the use of apple cider vinegar with a health professional.

There is also the possibility of apple cider vinegar interfering with correct working of diuretics and laxatives as well as drugs used to treat heart disease and diabetes. If you are prescribed drugs for any of these conditions you should seek advice from your doctor before using apple cider vinegar. Another problem with apple cider vinegar is that it can contain chromium which can have an effect on insulin levels in the body. This could be a concern for people with diabetes. The chromium is in the vinegar because apple trees naturally absorb this mineral and deposit it in the apple fruit. Because chromium improves insulin sensitivity it could actually be of use in treating diabetes, however, when used it on its own chromium is always used under medical supervision

Conclusion

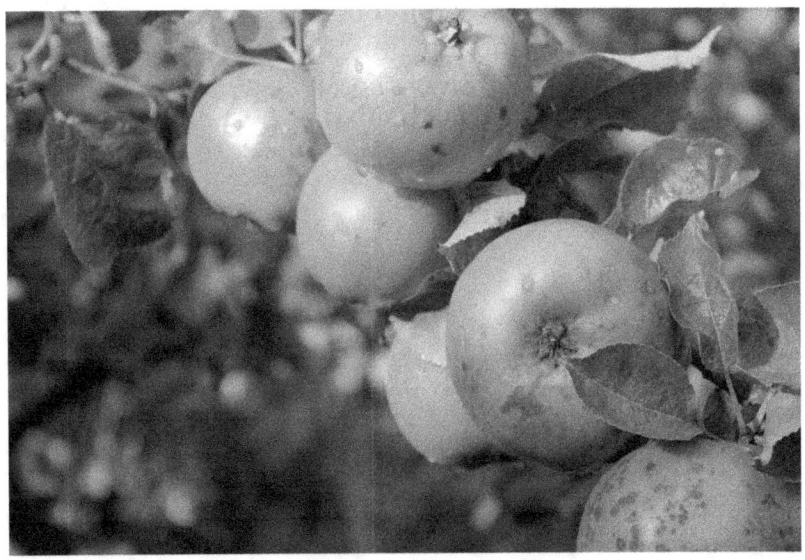

To get the most from apple cider vinegar make sure that you use the raw version rather than that which is processed and pasteurized. Raw apple cider vinegar contains far more useful natural products from both the cider itself and the vinegar production process.

It is cheaper to buy your apple cider vinegar straight from a farm where they make both the cider and the vinegar. We get ours from a fruit farm where they also grow the apples used. We therefore know that we are getting a completely natural product and we know its origins.

Try to use the vinegar in your cooking. There are plenty of recipes which include vinegar as one of the ingredients and there are also numerous salad dressings as well. You could also revive the pickling process and produce jars of pickled onions, garlic, chilies, beetroot, red cabbage and even wild mushrooms.

Apple cider vinegar is just one thing in a whole armory of natural treatments that can be tried. After using it you might like to look at such things as green smoothies, Rooibos tea, coconut oil and wheat grass as both supplements and as things that just generally enhance you diet and lifestyle.

About the Author

This book about the benefits of using Apple Cider Vinegar quickly followed Ellen Vincent's previous book called 'Green Smoothie'. Ellen uses both green smoothies and apple cider vinegar in her daily routine. Whereas green smoothies are only taken internally apple cider vinegar has the added benefit that it can be applied outside the body to the skin and hair. Rather than being considered as an alternative to green smoothies Ellen uses them together as part of her diet and for her skin and hair care as well. The two are complementary. As a result if you are already heavily involved in green smoothies you should also take a look at the benefits of Apple Cider Vinegar and vice versa. Apple Cider Vinegar is another completely natural product that allows you to stop using all of those artificial man made products that really don't help us at all.

Ellen has seen at first hand the differences that whole natural foods can make compared to the pre-packaged, processed and sanitized food that we eat in the west. In her native Ghana food comes straight from the field and is prepared in traditional ways.

Since living in the West she has sought to avoid the new processed foods that were presented to her and has embraced more natural diets. Apple cider vinegar and Green smoothies provide an excellent way of bringing these natural ways back into your life. She has found that there are great benefits to be gained from consuming the raw foods included in green smoothies and apple cider vinegar. After experiencing better health of body and mind from green smoothies and apple cider vinegar she was determined to show the rest of the world how they too could gain a better and healthier lifestyle.

Ellen is also interested in the natural care of hair and skin. She produces her own skin and hair care products from natural ingredients. These products have proved to be very successful and she is determined to produce a further book to show how these products can be combined with the benefits of green smoothies and apple cider vinegar to produce a complete system where skin and hair are kept in perfect condition by conditioning them from both the inside and outside of the body.

When thinking about our health and well being, you have to consider the fact that we really don't understand how all these modern chemical additives and treatments are affecting the human body. In the future people may look back in horror at what we have managed to do to ourselves, in much the same way that we view the use of poisons such as arsenic and red lead in cosmetics in the past. The best thing to do is to stick to the healthy options that come from the plants around us. Use the shea butter, coconut oils and other natural products because they have served us well for thousand of years and have never let us down. In all things, nature and not necessarily science and technology seems to know what is best for us.

www.ingramcontent.com/pod-product-compliance
Lightning Source LLC
Chambersburg PA
CBHW072332290526
45794CB00002B/847